Personal Data

Name ——————————————————
Phone ——————————————————
Adress ——————————————————

In case of emergency
Please contavt

Name ——————————————————
Phone ——————————————————
Adress ——————————————————

Essential Contacts

Doctor ——————————————————
Pharmacy ——————————————————
Eye Clinic ——————————————————
Dentist ——————————————————

Name ——————————————
Cell: ——————————————
Work: ——————————————
Home: ——————————————
Email: ——————————————
Others: ——————————————

Name ——————————————
Cell: ——————————————
Work: ——————————————
Home: ——————————————
Email: ——————————————
Others: ——————————————

Name ——————————————
Cell: ——————————————
Work: ——————————————
Home: ——————————————
Email: ——————————————
Others: ——————————————

Name ——————————————
Cell: ——————————————
Work: ——————————————
Home: ——————————————
Email: ——————————————
Others: ——————————————

Notes

Notes

Notes

Weekly Blood Sugar Log

Week_____

	Time	Before	After	Notes
Monday	Breakfast			
	Lunch			
	Dinner			
	Bedtime			
Tuesday	Breakfast			
	Lunch			
	Dinner			
	Bedtime			
Wednesday	Breakfast			
	Lunch			
	Dinner			
	Bedtime			
Thursday	Breakfast			
	Lunch			
	Dinner			
	Bedtime			
Friday	Breakfast			
	Lunch			
	Dinner			
	Bedtime			
Saturday	Breakfast			
	Lunch			
	Dinner			
	Bedtime			
Sunday	Breakfast			
	Lunch			
	Dinner			
	Bedtime			

Additional Notes

_____

_____

_____

_____

_____

Weekly Blood Sugar Log

Week_____

	Time	Before	After	Notes
Monday	Breakfast			
	Lunch			
	Dinner			
	Bedtime			
Tuesday	Breakfast			
	Lunch			
	Dinner			
	Bedtime			
Wednesday	Breakfast			
	Lunch			
	Dinner			
	Bedtime			
Thursday	Breakfast			
	Lunch			
	Dinner			
	Bedtime			
Friday	Breakfast			
	Lunch			
	Dinner			
	Bedtime			
Saturday	Breakfast			
	Lunch			
	Dinner			
	Bedtime			
Sunday	Breakfast			
	Lunch			
	Dinner			
	Bedtime			

Additional Notes

_____

_____

_____

_____

_____

Weekly Blood Sugar Log

Week_____

	Time	Before	After	Notes
Monday	Breakfast			
	Lunch			
	Dinner			
	Bedtime			
Tuesday	Breakfast			
	Lunch			
	Dinner			
	Bedtime			
Wednesday	Breakfast			
	Lunch			
	Dinner			
	Bedtime			
Thursday	Breakfast			
	Lunch			
	Dinner			
	Bedtime			
Friday	Breakfast			
	Lunch			
	Dinner			
	Bedtime			
Saturday	Breakfast			
	Lunch			
	Dinner			
	Bedtime			
Sunday	Breakfast			
	Lunch			
	Dinner			
	Bedtime			

Additional Notes

Weekly Blood Sugar Log

Week_____

	Time	Before	After	Notes
Monday	Breakfast			
	Lunch			
	Dinner			
	Bedtime			
Tuesday	Breakfast			
	Lunch			
	Dinner			
	Bedtime			
Wednesday	Breakfast			
	Lunch			
	Dinner			
	Bedtime			
Thursday	Breakfast			
	Lunch			
	Dinner			
	Bedtime			
Friday	Breakfast			
	Lunch			
	Dinner			
	Bedtime			
Saturday	Breakfast			
	Lunch			
	Dinner			
	Bedtime			
Sunday	Breakfast			
	Lunch			
	Dinner			
	Bedtime			

Additional Notes

_____

_____

_____

_____

_____

Weekly Blood Sugar Log

Week_____

	Time	Before	After	Notes
Monday	Breakfast			
	Lunch			
	Dinner			
	Bedtime			
Tuesday	Breakfast			
	Lunch			
	Dinner			
	Bedtime			
Wednesday	Breakfast			
	Lunch			
	Dinner			
	Bedtime			
Thursday	Breakfast			
	Lunch			
	Dinner			
	Bedtime			
Friday	Breakfast			
	Lunch			
	Dinner			
	Bedtime			
Saturday	Breakfast			
	Lunch			
	Dinner			
	Bedtime			
Sunday	Breakfast			
	Lunch			
	Dinner			
	Bedtime			

Additional Notes

_____

_____

_____

_____

_____

Weekly Blood Sugar Log

Week_____

	Time	Before	After	Notes
Monday	Breakfast			
	Lunch			
	Dinner			
	Bedtime			
Tuesday	Breakfast			
	Lunch			
	Dinner			
	Bedtime			
Wednesday	Breakfast			
	Lunch			
	Dinner			
	Bedtime			
Thursday	Breakfast			
	Lunch			
	Dinner			
	Bedtime			
Friday	Breakfast			
	Lunch			
	Dinner			
	Bedtime			
Saturday	Breakfast			
	Lunch			
	Dinner			
	Bedtime			
Sunday	Breakfast			
	Lunch			
	Dinner			
	Bedtime			

Additional Notes

Weekly Blood Sugar Log

Week_____

	Time	Before	After	Notes
Monday	Breakfast			
	Lunch			
	Dinner			
	Bedtime			
Tuesday	Breakfast			
	Lunch			
	Dinner			
	Bedtime			
Wednesday	Breakfast			
	Lunch			
	Dinner			
	Bedtime			
Thursday	Breakfast			
	Lunch			
	Dinner			
	Bedtime			
Friday	Breakfast			
	Lunch			
	Dinner			
	Bedtime			
Saturday	Breakfast			
	Lunch			
	Dinner			
	Bedtime			
Sunday	Breakfast			
	Lunch			
	Dinner			
	Bedtime			

Additional Notes

_____
_____
_____
_____
_____

Weekly Blood Sugar Log

Week_____

	Time	Before	After	Notes
Monday	Breakfast			
	Lunch			
	Dinner			
	Bedtime			
Tuesday	Breakfast			
	Lunch			
	Dinner			
	Bedtime			
Wednesday	Breakfast			
	Lunch			
	Dinner			
	Bedtime			
Thursday	Breakfast			
	Lunch			
	Dinner			
	Bedtime			
Friday	Breakfast			
	Lunch			
	Dinner			
	Bedtime			
Saturday	Breakfast			
	Lunch			
	Dinner			
	Bedtime			
Sunday	Breakfast			
	Lunch			
	Dinner			
	Bedtime			

Additional Notes

_____

_____

_____

_____

_____

Weekly Blood Sugar Log

Week_____

	Time	Before	After	Notes
Monday	Breakfast			
	Lunch			
	Dinner			
	Bedtime			
Tuesday	Breakfast			
	Lunch			
	Dinner			
	Bedtime			
Wednesday	Breakfast			
	Lunch			
	Dinner			
	Bedtime			
Thursday	Breakfast			
	Lunch			
	Dinner			
	Bedtime			
Friday	Breakfast			
	Lunch			
	Dinner			
	Bedtime			
Saturday	Breakfast			
	Lunch			
	Dinner			
	Bedtime			
Sunday	Breakfast			
	Lunch			
	Dinner			
	Bedtime			

Additional Notes

_____

_____

_____

_____

_____

Weekly Blood Sugar Log

Week_____

	Time	Before	After	Notes
Monday	Breakfast			
	Lunch			
	Dinner			
	Bedtime			
Tuesday	Breakfast			
	Lunch			
	Dinner			
	Bedtime			
Wednesday	Breakfast			
	Lunch			
	Dinner			
	Bedtime			
Thursday	Breakfast			
	Lunch			
	Dinner			
	Bedtime			
Friday	Breakfast			
	Lunch			
	Dinner			
	Bedtime			
Saturday	Breakfast			
	Lunch			
	Dinner			
	Bedtime			
Sunday	Breakfast			
	Lunch			
	Dinner			
	Bedtime			

Additional Notes

_____

_____

_____

_____

_____

Weekly Blood Sugar Log

Week_____

	Time	Before	After	Notes
Monday	Breakfast			
	Lunch			
	Dinner			
	Bedtime			
Tuesday	Breakfast			
	Lunch			
	Dinner			
	Bedtime			
Wednesday	Breakfast			
	Lunch			
	Dinner			
	Bedtime			
Thursday	Breakfast			
	Lunch			
	Dinner			
	Bedtime			
Friday	Breakfast			
	Lunch			
	Dinner			
	Bedtime			
Saturday	Breakfast			
	Lunch			
	Dinner			
	Bedtime			
Sunday	Breakfast			
	Lunch			
	Dinner			
	Bedtime			

Additional Notes

_____
_____
_____
_____
_____

Weekly Blood Sugar Log

Week_____

	Time	Before	After	Notes
Monday	Breakfast			
	Lunch			
	Dinner			
	Bedtime			
Tuesday	Breakfast			
	Lunch			
	Dinner			
	Bedtime			
Wednesday	Breakfast			
	Lunch			
	Dinner			
	Bedtime			
Thursday	Breakfast			
	Lunch			
	Dinner			
	Bedtime			
Friday	Breakfast			
	Lunch			
	Dinner			
	Bedtime			
Saturday	Breakfast			
	Lunch			
	Dinner			
	Bedtime			
Sunday	Breakfast			
	Lunch			
	Dinner			
	Bedtime			

Additional Notes

_____
_____
_____
_____
_____

Weekly Blood Sugar Log

Week_____

	Time	Before	After	Notes
Monday	Breakfast			
	Lunch			
	Dinner			
	Bedtime			
Tuesday	Breakfast			
	Lunch			
	Dinner			
	Bedtime			
Wednesday	Breakfast			
	Lunch			
	Dinner			
	Bedtime			
Thursday	Breakfast			
	Lunch			
	Dinner			
	Bedtime			
Friday	Breakfast			
	Lunch			
	Dinner			
	Bedtime			
Saturday	Breakfast			
	Lunch			
	Dinner			
	Bedtime			
Sunday	Breakfast			
	Lunch			
	Dinner			
	Bedtime			

Additional Notes

_____
_____
_____
_____
_____

Weekly Blood Sugar Log

Week_____

	Time	Before	After	Notes
Monday	Breakfast			
	Lunch			
	Dinner			
	Bedtime			
Tuesday	Breakfast			
	Lunch			
	Dinner			
	Bedtime			
Wednesday	Breakfast			
	Lunch			
	Dinner			
	Bedtime			
Thursday	Breakfast			
	Lunch			
	Dinner			
	Bedtime			
Friday	Breakfast			
	Lunch			
	Dinner			
	Bedtime			
Saturday	Breakfast			
	Lunch			
	Dinner			
	Bedtime			
Sunday	Breakfast			
	Lunch			
	Dinner			
	Bedtime			

Additional Notes

_____

_____

_____

_____

_____

Weekly Blood Sugar Log

Week_____

	Time	Before	After	Notes
Monday	Breakfast			
	Lunch			
	Dinner			
	Bedtime			
Tuesday	Breakfast			
	Lunch			
	Dinner			
	Bedtime			
Wednesday	Breakfast			
	Lunch			
	Dinner			
	Bedtime			
Thursday	Breakfast			
	Lunch			
	Dinner			
	Bedtime			
Friday	Breakfast			
	Lunch			
	Dinner			
	Bedtime			
Saturday	Breakfast			
	Lunch			
	Dinner			
	Bedtime			
Sunday	Breakfast			
	Lunch			
	Dinner			
	Bedtime			

Additional Notes

_____
_____
_____
_____
_____

Weekly Blood Sugar Log

Week_____

	Time	Before	After	Notes
Monday	Breakfast			
	Lunch			
	Dinner			
	Bedtime			
Tuesday	Breakfast			
	Lunch			
	Dinner			
	Bedtime			
Wednesday	Breakfast			
	Lunch			
	Dinner			
	Bedtime			
Thursday	Breakfast			
	Lunch			
	Dinner			
	Bedtime			
Friday	Breakfast			
	Lunch			
	Dinner			
	Bedtime			
Saturday	Breakfast			
	Lunch			
	Dinner			
	Bedtime			
Sunday	Breakfast			
	Lunch			
	Dinner			
	Bedtime			

Additional Notes

_____
_____
_____
_____
_____

Weekly Blood Sugar Log

Week_____

	Time	Before	After	Notes
Monday	Breakfast			
	Lunch			
	Dinner			
	Bedtime			
Tuesday	Breakfast			
	Lunch			
	Dinner			
	Bedtime			
Wednesday	Breakfast			
	Lunch			
	Dinner			
	Bedtime			
Thursday	Breakfast			
	Lunch			
	Dinner			
	Bedtime			
Friday	Breakfast			
	Lunch			
	Dinner			
	Bedtime			
Saturday	Breakfast			
	Lunch			
	Dinner			
	Bedtime			
Sunday	Breakfast			
	Lunch			
	Dinner			
	Bedtime			

Additional Notes

Weekly Blood Sugar Log

Week_____

	Time	Before	After	Notes
Monday	Breakfast			
	Lunch			
	Dinner			
	Bedtime			
Tuesday	Breakfast			
	Lunch			
	Dinner			
	Bedtime			
Wednesday	Breakfast			
	Lunch			
	Dinner			
	Bedtime			
Thursday	Breakfast			
	Lunch			
	Dinner			
	Bedtime			
Friday	Breakfast			
	Lunch			
	Dinner			
	Bedtime			
Saturday	Breakfast			
	Lunch			
	Dinner			
	Bedtime			
Sunday	Breakfast			
	Lunch			
	Dinner			
	Bedtime			

Additional Notes

_____
_____
_____
_____
_____

Weekly Blood Sugar Log

Week_____

	Time	Before	After	Notes
Monday	Breakfast			
	Lunch			
	Dinner			
	Bedtime			
Tuesday	Breakfast			
	Lunch			
	Dinner			
	Bedtime			
Wednesday	Breakfast			
	Lunch			
	Dinner			
	Bedtime			
Thursday	Breakfast			
	Lunch			
	Dinner			
	Bedtime			
Friday	Breakfast			
	Lunch			
	Dinner			
	Bedtime			
Saturday	Breakfast			
	Lunch			
	Dinner			
	Bedtime			
Sunday	Breakfast			
	Lunch			
	Dinner			
	Bedtime			

Additional Notes

_____

_____

_____

_____

_____

Weekly Blood Sugar Log

Week_____

	Time	Before	After	Notes
Monday	Breakfast			
	Lunch			
	Dinner			
	Bedtime			
Tuesday	Breakfast			
	Lunch			
	Dinner			
	Bedtime			
Wednesday	Breakfast			
	Lunch			
	Dinner			
	Bedtime			
Thursday	Breakfast			
	Lunch			
	Dinner			
	Bedtime			
Friday	Breakfast			
	Lunch			
	Dinner			
	Bedtime			
Saturday	Breakfast			
	Lunch			
	Dinner			
	Bedtime			
Sunday	Breakfast			
	Lunch			
	Dinner			
	Bedtime			

Additional Notes

_____

_____

_____

_____

_____

Weekly Blood Sugar Log

Week_____

	Time	Before	After	Notes
Monday	Breakfast			
	Lunch			
	Dinner			
	Bedtime			
Tuesday	Breakfast			
	Lunch			
	Dinner			
	Bedtime			
Wednesday	Breakfast			
	Lunch			
	Dinner			
	Bedtime			
Thursday	Breakfast			
	Lunch			
	Dinner			
	Bedtime			
Friday	Breakfast			
	Lunch			
	Dinner			
	Bedtime			
Saturday	Breakfast			
	Lunch			
	Dinner			
	Bedtime			
Sunday	Breakfast			
	Lunch			
	Dinner			
	Bedtime			

Additional Notes

_____

_____

_____

_____

_____

Weekly Blood Sugar Log

Week_____

	Time	Before	After	Notes
Monday	Breakfast			
	Lunch			
	Dinner			
	Bedtime			
Tuesday	Breakfast			
	Lunch			
	Dinner			
	Bedtime			
Wednesday	Breakfast			
	Lunch			
	Dinner			
	Bedtime			
Thursday	Breakfast			
	Lunch			
	Dinner			
	Bedtime			
Friday	Breakfast			
	Lunch			
	Dinner			
	Bedtime			
Saturday	Breakfast			
	Lunch			
	Dinner			
	Bedtime			
Sunday	Breakfast			
	Lunch			
	Dinner			
	Bedtime			

Additional Notes

_____
_____
_____
_____
_____

Weekly Blood Sugar Log

Week_____

	Time	Before	After	Notes
Monday	Breakfast			
	Lunch			
	Dinner			
	Bedtime			
Tuesday	Breakfast			
	Lunch			
	Dinner			
	Bedtime			
Wednesday	Breakfast			
	Lunch			
	Dinner			
	Bedtime			
Thursday	Breakfast			
	Lunch			
	Dinner			
	Bedtime			
Friday	Breakfast			
	Lunch			
	Dinner			
	Bedtime			
Saturday	Breakfast			
	Lunch			
	Dinner			
	Bedtime			
Sunday	Breakfast			
	Lunch			
	Dinner			
	Bedtime			

Additional Notes

_____

_____

_____

_____

_____

Weekly Blood Sugar Log

Week_____

	Time	Before	After	Notes
Monday	Breakfast			
	Lunch			
	Dinner			
	Bedtime			
Tuesday	Breakfast			
	Lunch			
	Dinner			
	Bedtime			
Wednesday	Breakfast			
	Lunch			
	Dinner			
	Bedtime			
Thursday	Breakfast			
	Lunch			
	Dinner			
	Bedtime			
Friday	Breakfast			
	Lunch			
	Dinner			
	Bedtime			
Saturday	Breakfast			
	Lunch			
	Dinner			
	Bedtime			
Sunday	Breakfast			
	Lunch			
	Dinner			
	Bedtime			

Additional Notes

_____

_____

_____

_____

_____

Weekly Blood Sugar Log

Week_____

	Time	Before	After	Notes
Monday	Breakfast			
	Lunch			
	Dinner			
	Bedtime			
Tuesday	Breakfast			
	Lunch			
	Dinner			
	Bedtime			
Wednesday	Breakfast			
	Lunch			
	Dinner			
	Bedtime			
Thursday	Breakfast			
	Lunch			
	Dinner			
	Bedtime			
Friday	Breakfast			
	Lunch			
	Dinner			
	Bedtime			
Saturday	Breakfast			
	Lunch			
	Dinner			
	Bedtime			
Sunday	Breakfast			
	Lunch			
	Dinner			
	Bedtime			

Additional Notes

_____

_____

_____

_____

_____

Weekly Blood Sugar Log

Week_____

	Time	Before	After	Notes
Monday	Breakfast			
	Lunch			
	Dinner			
	Bedtime			
Tuesday	Breakfast			
	Lunch			
	Dinner			
	Bedtime			
Wednesday	Breakfast			
	Lunch			
	Dinner			
	Bedtime			
Thursday	Breakfast			
	Lunch			
	Dinner			
	Bedtime			
Friday	Breakfast			
	Lunch			
	Dinner			
	Bedtime			
Saturday	Breakfast			
	Lunch			
	Dinner			
	Bedtime			
Sunday	Breakfast			
	Lunch			
	Dinner			
	Bedtime			

Additional Notes

_____

_____

_____

_____

_____

Weekly Blood Sugar Log

Week_____

	Time	Before	After	Notes
Monday	Breakfast			
	Lunch			
	Dinner			
	Bedtime			
Tuesday	Breakfast			
	Lunch			
	Dinner			
	Bedtime			
Wednesday	Breakfast			
	Lunch			
	Dinner			
	Bedtime			
Thursday	Breakfast			
	Lunch			
	Dinner			
	Bedtime			
Friday	Breakfast			
	Lunch			
	Dinner			
	Bedtime			
Saturday	Breakfast			
	Lunch			
	Dinner			
	Bedtime			
Sunday	Breakfast			
	Lunch			
	Dinner			
	Bedtime			

Additional Notes

_____
_____
_____
_____
_____

Weekly Blood Sugar Log

Week_____

	Time	Before	After	Notes
Monday	Breakfast			
	Lunch			
	Dinner			
	Bedtime			
Tuesday	Breakfast			
	Lunch			
	Dinner			
	Bedtime			
Wednesday	Breakfast			
	Lunch			
	Dinner			
	Bedtime			
Thursday	Breakfast			
	Lunch			
	Dinner			
	Bedtime			
Friday	Breakfast			
	Lunch			
	Dinner			
	Bedtime			
Saturday	Breakfast			
	Lunch			
	Dinner			
	Bedtime			
Sunday	Breakfast			
	Lunch			
	Dinner			
	Bedtime			

Additional Notes

_____
_____
_____
_____
_____

Weekly Blood Sugar Log

Week_____

	Time	Before	After	Notes
Monday	Breakfast			
	Lunch			
	Dinner			
	Bedtime			
Tuesday	Breakfast			
	Lunch			
	Dinner			
	Bedtime			
Wednesday	Breakfast			
	Lunch			
	Dinner			
	Bedtime			
Thursday	Breakfast			
	Lunch			
	Dinner			
	Bedtime			
Friday	Breakfast			
	Lunch			
	Dinner			
	Bedtime			
Saturday	Breakfast			
	Lunch			
	Dinner			
	Bedtime			
Sunday	Breakfast			
	Lunch			
	Dinner			
	Bedtime			

Additional Notes

Weekly Blood Sugar Log

Week_____

	Time	Before	After	Notes
Monday	Breakfast			
	Lunch			
	Dinner			
	Bedtime			
Tuesday	Breakfast			
	Lunch			
	Dinner			
	Bedtime			
Wednesday	Breakfast			
	Lunch			
	Dinner			
	Bedtime			
Thursday	Breakfast			
	Lunch			
	Dinner			
	Bedtime			
Friday	Breakfast			
	Lunch			
	Dinner			
	Bedtime			
Saturday	Breakfast			
	Lunch			
	Dinner			
	Bedtime			
Sunday	Breakfast			
	Lunch			
	Dinner			
	Bedtime			

Additional Notes

_____

_____

_____

_____

_____

Weekly Blood Sugar Log

Week_____

	Time	Before	After	Notes
Monday	Breakfast			
	Lunch			
	Dinner			
	Bedtime			
Tuesday	Breakfast			
	Lunch			
	Dinner			
	Bedtime			
Wednesday	Breakfast			
	Lunch			
	Dinner			
	Bedtime			
Thursday	Breakfast			
	Lunch			
	Dinner			
	Bedtime			
Friday	Breakfast			
	Lunch			
	Dinner			
	Bedtime			
Saturday	Breakfast			
	Lunch			
	Dinner			
	Bedtime			
Sunday	Breakfast			
	Lunch			
	Dinner			
	Bedtime			

Additional Notes

_____
_____
_____
_____
_____

Weekly Blood Sugar Log

Week_____

	Time	Before	After	Notes
Monday	Breakfast			
	Lunch			
	Dinner			
	Bedtime			
Tuesday	Breakfast			
	Lunch			
	Dinner			
	Bedtime			
Wednesday	Breakfast			
	Lunch			
	Dinner			
	Bedtime			
Thursday	Breakfast			
	Lunch			
	Dinner			
	Bedtime			
Friday	Breakfast			
	Lunch			
	Dinner			
	Bedtime			
Saturday	Breakfast			
	Lunch			
	Dinner			
	Bedtime			
Sunday	Breakfast			
	Lunch			
	Dinner			
	Bedtime			

Additional Notes

_____

_____

_____

_____

_____

Weekly Blood Sugar Log

Week_____

	Time	Before	After	Notes
Monday	Breakfast			
	Lunch			
	Dinner			
	Bedtime			
Tuesday	Breakfast			
	Lunch			
	Dinner			
	Bedtime			
Wednesday	Breakfast			
	Lunch			
	Dinner			
	Bedtime			
Thursday	Breakfast			
	Lunch			
	Dinner			
	Bedtime			
Friday	Breakfast			
	Lunch			
	Dinner			
	Bedtime			
Saturday	Breakfast			
	Lunch			
	Dinner			
	Bedtime			
Sunday	Breakfast			
	Lunch			
	Dinner			
	Bedtime			

Additional Notes

_____

_____

_____

_____

_____

Weekly Blood Sugar Log

Week_____

	Time	Before	After	Notes
Monday	Breakfast			
	Lunch			
	Dinner			
	Bedtime			
Tuesday	Breakfast			
	Lunch			
	Dinner			
	Bedtime			
Wednesday	Breakfast			
	Lunch			
	Dinner			
	Bedtime			
Thursday	Breakfast			
	Lunch			
	Dinner			
	Bedtime			
Friday	Breakfast			
	Lunch			
	Dinner			
	Bedtime			
Saturday	Breakfast			
	Lunch			
	Dinner			
	Bedtime			
Sunday	Breakfast			
	Lunch			
	Dinner			
	Bedtime			

Additional Notes

_____

_____

_____

_____

_____

Weekly Blood Sugar Log

Week_____

	Time	Before	After	Notes
Monday	Breakfast			
	Lunch			
	Dinner			
	Bedtime			
Tuesday	Breakfast			
	Lunch			
	Dinner			
	Bedtime			
Wednesday	Breakfast			
	Lunch			
	Dinner			
	Bedtime			
Thursday	Breakfast			
	Lunch			
	Dinner			
	Bedtime			
Friday	Breakfast			
	Lunch			
	Dinner			
	Bedtime			
Saturday	Breakfast			
	Lunch			
	Dinner			
	Bedtime			
Sunday	Breakfast			
	Lunch			
	Dinner			
	Bedtime			

Additional Notes

_____

_____

_____

_____

_____

Weekly Blood Sugar Log

Week_____

	Time	Before	After	Notes
Monday	Breakfast			
	Lunch			
	Dinner			
	Bedtime			
Tuesday	Breakfast			
	Lunch			
	Dinner			
	Bedtime			
Wednesday	Breakfast			
	Lunch			
	Dinner			
	Bedtime			
Thursday	Breakfast			
	Lunch			
	Dinner			
	Bedtime			
Friday	Breakfast			
	Lunch			
	Dinner			
	Bedtime			
Saturday	Breakfast			
	Lunch			
	Dinner			
	Bedtime			
Sunday	Breakfast			
	Lunch			
	Dinner			
	Bedtime			

Additional Notes

_____

_____

_____

_____

_____

Weekly Blood Sugar Log

Week_____

	Time	Before	After	Notes
Monday	Breakfast			
	Lunch			
	Dinner			
	Bedtime			
Tuesday	Breakfast			
	Lunch			
	Dinner			
	Bedtime			
Wednesday	Breakfast			
	Lunch			
	Dinner			
	Bedtime			
Thursday	Breakfast			
	Lunch			
	Dinner			
	Bedtime			
Friday	Breakfast			
	Lunch			
	Dinner			
	Bedtime			
Saturday	Breakfast			
	Lunch			
	Dinner			
	Bedtime			
Sunday	Breakfast			
	Lunch			
	Dinner			
	Bedtime			

Additional Notes

_____
_____
_____
_____
_____

Weekly Blood Sugar Log

Week_____

	Time	Before	After	Notes
Monday	Breakfast			
	Lunch			
	Dinner			
	Bedtime			
Tuesday	Breakfast			
	Lunch			
	Dinner			
	Bedtime			
Wednesday	Breakfast			
	Lunch			
	Dinner			
	Bedtime			
Thursday	Breakfast			
	Lunch			
	Dinner			
	Bedtime			
Friday	Breakfast			
	Lunch			
	Dinner			
	Bedtime			
Saturday	Breakfast			
	Lunch			
	Dinner			
	Bedtime			
Sunday	Breakfast			
	Lunch			
	Dinner			
	Bedtime			

Additional Notes

_____
_____
_____
_____
_____

Weekly Blood Sugar Log

Week_____

	Time	Before	After	Notes
Monday	Breakfast			
	Lunch			
	Dinner			
	Bedtime			
Tuesday	Breakfast			
	Lunch			
	Dinner			
	Bedtime			
Wednesday	Breakfast			
	Lunch			
	Dinner			
	Bedtime			
Thursday	Breakfast			
	Lunch			
	Dinner			
	Bedtime			
Friday	Breakfast			
	Lunch			
	Dinner			
	Bedtime			
Saturday	Breakfast			
	Lunch			
	Dinner			
	Bedtime			
Sunday	Breakfast			
	Lunch			
	Dinner			
	Bedtime			

Additional Notes

_____
_____
_____
_____
_____

Weekly Blood Sugar Log

Week_____

	Time	Before	After	Notes
Monday	Breakfast			
	Lunch			
	Dinner			
	Bedtime			
Tuesday	Breakfast			
	Lunch			
	Dinner			
	Bedtime			
Wednesday	Breakfast			
	Lunch			
	Dinner			
	Bedtime			
Thursday	Breakfast			
	Lunch			
	Dinner			
	Bedtime			
Friday	Breakfast			
	Lunch			
	Dinner			
	Bedtime			
Saturday	Breakfast			
	Lunch			
	Dinner			
	Bedtime			
Sunday	Breakfast			
	Lunch			
	Dinner			
	Bedtime			

Additional Notes

Weekly Blood Sugar Log

Week_____

	Time	Before	After	Notes
Monday	Breakfast			
	Lunch			
	Dinner			
	Bedtime			
Tuesday	Breakfast			
	Lunch			
	Dinner			
	Bedtime			
Wednesday	Breakfast			
	Lunch			
	Dinner			
	Bedtime			
Thursday	Breakfast			
	Lunch			
	Dinner			
	Bedtime			
Friday	Breakfast			
	Lunch			
	Dinner			
	Bedtime			
Saturday	Breakfast			
	Lunch			
	Dinner			
	Bedtime			
Sunday	Breakfast			
	Lunch			
	Dinner			
	Bedtime			

Additional Notes

_____
_____
_____
_____
_____

Weekly Blood Sugar Log

Week_____

	Time	Before	After	Notes
Monday	Breakfast			
	Lunch			
	Dinner			
	Bedtime			
Tuesday	Breakfast			
	Lunch			
	Dinner			
	Bedtime			
Wednesday	Breakfast			
	Lunch			
	Dinner			
	Bedtime			
Thursday	Breakfast			
	Lunch			
	Dinner			
	Bedtime			
Friday	Breakfast			
	Lunch			
	Dinner			
	Bedtime			
Saturday	Breakfast			
	Lunch			
	Dinner			
	Bedtime			
Sunday	Breakfast			
	Lunch			
	Dinner			
	Bedtime			

Additional Notes

_____
_____
_____
_____
_____

Weekly Blood Sugar Log

Week_____

	Time	Before	After	Notes
Monday	Breakfast			
	Lunch			
	Dinner			
	Bedtime			
Tuesday	Breakfast			
	Lunch			
	Dinner			
	Bedtime			
Wednesday	Breakfast			
	Lunch			
	Dinner			
	Bedtime			
Thursday	Breakfast			
	Lunch			
	Dinner			
	Bedtime			
Friday	Breakfast			
	Lunch			
	Dinner			
	Bedtime			
Saturday	Breakfast			
	Lunch			
	Dinner			
	Bedtime			
Sunday	Breakfast			
	Lunch			
	Dinner			
	Bedtime			

Additional Notes

_____

_____

_____

_____

_____

Weekly Blood Sugar Log

Week_____

	Time	Before	After	Notes
Monday	Breakfast			
	Lunch			
	Dinner			
	Bedtime			
Tuesday	Breakfast			
	Lunch			
	Dinner			
	Bedtime			
Wednesday	Breakfast			
	Lunch			
	Dinner			
	Bedtime			
Thursday	Breakfast			
	Lunch			
	Dinner			
	Bedtime			
Friday	Breakfast			
	Lunch			
	Dinner			
	Bedtime			
Saturday	Breakfast			
	Lunch			
	Dinner			
	Bedtime			
Sunday	Breakfast			
	Lunch			
	Dinner			
	Bedtime			

Additional Notes

_____

_____

_____

_____

_____

Weekly Blood Sugar Log

Week_____

	Time	Before	After	Notes
Monday	Breakfast			
	Lunch			
	Dinner			
	Bedtime			
Tuesday	Breakfast			
	Lunch			
	Dinner			
	Bedtime			
Wednesday	Breakfast			
	Lunch			
	Dinner			
	Bedtime			
Thursday	Breakfast			
	Lunch			
	Dinner			
	Bedtime			
Friday	Breakfast			
	Lunch			
	Dinner			
	Bedtime			
Saturday	Breakfast			
	Lunch			
	Dinner			
	Bedtime			
Sunday	Breakfast			
	Lunch			
	Dinner			
	Bedtime			

Additional Notes

_____
_____
_____
_____
_____

Weekly Blood Sugar Log

Week_____

	Time	Before	After	Notes
Monday	Breakfast			
	Lunch			
	Dinner			
	Bedtime			
Tuesday	Breakfast			
	Lunch			
	Dinner			
	Bedtime			
Wednesday	Breakfast			
	Lunch			
	Dinner			
	Bedtime			
Thursday	Breakfast			
	Lunch			
	Dinner			
	Bedtime			
Friday	Breakfast			
	Lunch			
	Dinner			
	Bedtime			
Saturday	Breakfast			
	Lunch			
	Dinner			
	Bedtime			
Sunday	Breakfast			
	Lunch			
	Dinner			
	Bedtime			

Additional Notes

_____
_____
_____
_____
_____

Weekly Blood Sugar Log

Week_____

	Time	Before	After	Notes
Monday	Breakfast			
	Lunch			
	Dinner			
	Bedtime			
Tuesday	Breakfast			
	Lunch			
	Dinner			
	Bedtime			
Wednesday	Breakfast			
	Lunch			
	Dinner			
	Bedtime			
Thursday	Breakfast			
	Lunch			
	Dinner			
	Bedtime			
Friday	Breakfast			
	Lunch			
	Dinner			
	Bedtime			
Saturday	Breakfast			
	Lunch			
	Dinner			
	Bedtime			
Sunday	Breakfast			
	Lunch			
	Dinner			
	Bedtime			

Additional Notes

_____

_____

_____

_____

Weekly Blood Sugar Log

Week_____

	Time	Before	After	Notes
Monday	Breakfast			
	Lunch			
	Dinner			
	Bedtime			
Tuesday	Breakfast			
	Lunch			
	Dinner			
	Bedtime			
Wednesday	Breakfast			
	Lunch			
	Dinner			
	Bedtime			
Thursday	Breakfast			
	Lunch			
	Dinner			
	Bedtime			
Friday	Breakfast			
	Lunch			
	Dinner			
	Bedtime			
Saturday	Breakfast			
	Lunch			
	Dinner			
	Bedtime			
Sunday	Breakfast			
	Lunch			
	Dinner			
	Bedtime			

Additional Notes

_____

_____

_____

_____

_____

Weekly Blood Sugar Log

Week_____

	Time	Before	After	Notes
Monday	Breakfast			
	Lunch			
	Dinner			
	Bedtime			
Tuesday	Breakfast			
	Lunch			
	Dinner			
	Bedtime			
Wednesday	Breakfast			
	Lunch			
	Dinner			
	Bedtime			
Thursday	Breakfast			
	Lunch			
	Dinner			
	Bedtime			
Friday	Breakfast			
	Lunch			
	Dinner			
	Bedtime			
Saturday	Breakfast			
	Lunch			
	Dinner			
	Bedtime			
Sunday	Breakfast			
	Lunch			
	Dinner			
	Bedtime			

Additional Notes

_____

_____

_____

_____

_____

Weekly Blood Sugar Log

Week_____

	Time	Before	After	Notes
Monday	Breakfast			
	Lunch			
	Dinner			
	Bedtime			
Tuesday	Breakfast			
	Lunch			
	Dinner			
	Bedtime			
Wednesday	Breakfast			
	Lunch			
	Dinner			
	Bedtime			
Thursday	Breakfast			
	Lunch			
	Dinner			
	Bedtime			
Friday	Breakfast			
	Lunch			
	Dinner			
	Bedtime			
Saturday	Breakfast			
	Lunch			
	Dinner			
	Bedtime			
Sunday	Breakfast			
	Lunch			
	Dinner			
	Bedtime			

Additional Notes

_____

_____

_____

_____

_____

Weekly Blood Sugar Log

Week_____

	Time	Before	After	Notes
Monday	Breakfast			
	Lunch			
	Dinner			
	Bedtime			
Tuesday	Breakfast			
	Lunch			
	Dinner			
	Bedtime			
Wednesday	Breakfast			
	Lunch			
	Dinner			
	Bedtime			
Thursday	Breakfast			
	Lunch			
	Dinner			
	Bedtime			
Friday	Breakfast			
	Lunch			
	Dinner			
	Bedtime			
Saturday	Breakfast			
	Lunch			
	Dinner			
	Bedtime			
Sunday	Breakfast			
	Lunch			
	Dinner			
	Bedtime			

Additional Notes

_____

_____

_____

_____

_____

Weekly Blood Sugar Log

Week_____

	Time	Before	After	Notes
Monday	Breakfast			
	Lunch			
	Dinner			
	Bedtime			
Tuesday	Breakfast			
	Lunch			
	Dinner			
	Bedtime			
Wednesday	Breakfast			
	Lunch			
	Dinner			
	Bedtime			
Thursday	Breakfast			
	Lunch			
	Dinner			
	Bedtime			
Friday	Breakfast			
	Lunch			
	Dinner			
	Bedtime			
Saturday	Breakfast			
	Lunch			
	Dinner			
	Bedtime			
Sunday	Breakfast			
	Lunch			
	Dinner			
	Bedtime			

Additional Notes

_____

_____

_____

_____

_____

Weekly Blood Sugar Log

Week_____

	Time	Before	After	Notes
Monday	Breakfast			
	Lunch			
	Dinner			
	Bedtime			
Tuesday	Breakfast			
	Lunch			
	Dinner			
	Bedtime			
Wednesday	Breakfast			
	Lunch			
	Dinner			
	Bedtime			
Thursday	Breakfast			
	Lunch			
	Dinner			
	Bedtime			
Friday	Breakfast			
	Lunch			
	Dinner			
	Bedtime			
Saturday	Breakfast			
	Lunch			
	Dinner			
	Bedtime			
Sunday	Breakfast			
	Lunch			
	Dinner			
	Bedtime			

Additional Notes

_____

_____

_____

_____

_____

Weekly Blood Sugar Log

Week_____

	Time	Before	After	Notes
Monday	Breakfast			
	Lunch			
	Dinner			
	Bedtime			
Tuesday	Breakfast			
	Lunch			
	Dinner			
	Bedtime			
Wednesday	Breakfast			
	Lunch			
	Dinner			
	Bedtime			
Thursday	Breakfast			
	Lunch			
	Dinner			
	Bedtime			
Friday	Breakfast			
	Lunch			
	Dinner			
	Bedtime			
Saturday	Breakfast			
	Lunch			
	Dinner			
	Bedtime			
Sunday	Breakfast			
	Lunch			
	Dinner			
	Bedtime			

Additional Notes

_____

_____

_____

_____

_____

Weekly Blood Sugar Log

Week_____

	Time	Before	After	Notes
Monday	Breakfast			
	Lunch			
	Dinner			
	Bedtime			
Tuesday	Breakfast			
	Lunch			
	Dinner			
	Bedtime			
Wednesday	Breakfast			
	Lunch			
	Dinner			
	Bedtime			
Thursday	Breakfast			
	Lunch			
	Dinner			
	Bedtime			
Friday	Breakfast			
	Lunch			
	Dinner			
	Bedtime			
Saturday	Breakfast			
	Lunch			
	Dinner			
	Bedtime			
Sunday	Breakfast			
	Lunch			
	Dinner			
	Bedtime			

Additional Notes

_____

_____

_____

_____

_____

Weekly Blood Sugar Log

Week_____

	Time	Before	After	Notes
Monday	Breakfast			
	Lunch			
	Dinner			
	Bedtime			
Tuesday	Breakfast			
	Lunch			
	Dinner			
	Bedtime			
Wednesday	Breakfast			
	Lunch			
	Dinner			
	Bedtime			
Thursday	Breakfast			
	Lunch			
	Dinner			
	Bedtime			
Friday	Breakfast			
	Lunch			
	Dinner			
	Bedtime			
Saturday	Breakfast			
	Lunch			
	Dinner			
	Bedtime			
Sunday	Breakfast			
	Lunch			
	Dinner			
	Bedtime			

Additional Notes

_____
_____
_____
_____
_____

Weekly Blood Sugar Log

Week_____

	Time	Before	After	Notes
Monday	Breakfast			
	Lunch			
	Dinner			
	Bedtime			
Tuesday	Breakfast			
	Lunch			
	Dinner			
	Bedtime			
Wednesday	Breakfast			
	Lunch			
	Dinner			
	Bedtime			
Thursday	Breakfast			
	Lunch			
	Dinner			
	Bedtime			
Friday	Breakfast			
	Lunch			
	Dinner			
	Bedtime			
Saturday	Breakfast			
	Lunch			
	Dinner			
	Bedtime			
Sunday	Breakfast			
	Lunch			
	Dinner			
	Bedtime			

Additional Notes

Weekly Blood Sugar Log

Week_____

	Time	Before	After	Notes
Monday	Breakfast			
	Lunch			
	Dinner			
	Bedtime			
Tuesday	Breakfast			
	Lunch			
	Dinner			
	Bedtime			
Wednesday	Breakfast			
	Lunch			
	Dinner			
	Bedtime			
Thursday	Breakfast			
	Lunch			
	Dinner			
	Bedtime			
Friday	Breakfast			
	Lunch			
	Dinner			
	Bedtime			
Saturday	Breakfast			
	Lunch			
	Dinner			
	Bedtime			
Sunday	Breakfast			
	Lunch			
	Dinner			
	Bedtime			

Additional Notes

_____
_____
_____
_____
_____

Weekly Blood Sugar Log

Week_____

	Time	Before	After	Notes
Monday	Breakfast			
	Lunch			
	Dinner			
	Bedtime			
Tuesday	Breakfast			
	Lunch			
	Dinner			
	Bedtime			
Wednesday	Breakfast			
	Lunch			
	Dinner			
	Bedtime			
Thursday	Breakfast			
	Lunch			
	Dinner			
	Bedtime			
Friday	Breakfast			
	Lunch			
	Dinner			
	Bedtime			
Saturday	Breakfast			
	Lunch			
	Dinner			
	Bedtime			
Sunday	Breakfast			
	Lunch			
	Dinner			
	Bedtime			

Additional Notes

_____
_____
_____
_____
_____

Weekly Blood Sugar Log

Week_____

	Time	Before	After	Notes
Monday	Breakfast			
	Lunch			
	Dinner			
	Bedtime			
Tuesday	Breakfast			
	Lunch			
	Dinner			
	Bedtime			
Wednesday	Breakfast			
	Lunch			
	Dinner			
	Bedtime			
Thursday	Breakfast			
	Lunch			
	Dinner			
	Bedtime			
Friday	Breakfast			
	Lunch			
	Dinner			
	Bedtime			
Saturday	Breakfast			
	Lunch			
	Dinner			
	Bedtime			
Sunday	Breakfast			
	Lunch			
	Dinner			
	Bedtime			

Additional Notes

_____

_____

_____

_____

_____

Weekly Blood Sugar Log

Week_____

	Time	Before	After	Notes
Monday	Breakfast			
	Lunch			
	Dinner			
	Bedtime			
Tuesday	Breakfast			
	Lunch			
	Dinner			
	Bedtime			
Wednesday	Breakfast			
	Lunch			
	Dinner			
	Bedtime			
Thursday	Breakfast			
	Lunch			
	Dinner			
	Bedtime			
Friday	Breakfast			
	Lunch			
	Dinner			
	Bedtime			
Saturday	Breakfast			
	Lunch			
	Dinner			
	Bedtime			
Sunday	Breakfast			
	Lunch			
	Dinner			
	Bedtime			

Additional Notes

_____

_____

_____

_____

_____

Weekly Blood Sugar Log

Week_____

	Time	Before	After	Notes
Monday	Breakfast			
	Lunch			
	Dinner			
	Bedtime			
Tuesday	Breakfast			
	Lunch			
	Dinner			
	Bedtime			
Wednesday	Breakfast			
	Lunch			
	Dinner			
	Bedtime			
Thursday	Breakfast			
	Lunch			
	Dinner			
	Bedtime			
Friday	Breakfast			
	Lunch			
	Dinner			
	Bedtime			
Saturday	Breakfast			
	Lunch			
	Dinner			
	Bedtime			
Sunday	Breakfast			
	Lunch			
	Dinner			
	Bedtime			

Additional Notes

_____

_____

_____

_____

_____

Weekly Blood Sugar Log

Week_____

	Time	Before	After	Notes
Monday	Breakfast			
	Lunch			
	Dinner			
	Bedtime			
Tuesday	Breakfast			
	Lunch			
	Dinner			
	Bedtime			
Wednesday	Breakfast			
	Lunch			
	Dinner			
	Bedtime			
Thursday	Breakfast			
	Lunch			
	Dinner			
	Bedtime			
Friday	Breakfast			
	Lunch			
	Dinner			
	Bedtime			
Saturday	Breakfast			
	Lunch			
	Dinner			
	Bedtime			
Sunday	Breakfast			
	Lunch			
	Dinner			
	Bedtime			

Additional Notes

_____

_____

_____

_____

_____

Weekly Blood Sugar Log

Week_____

	Time	Before	After	Notes
Monday	Breakfast			
	Lunch			
	Dinner			
	Bedtime			
Tuesday	Breakfast			
	Lunch			
	Dinner			
	Bedtime			
Wednesday	Breakfast			
	Lunch			
	Dinner			
	Bedtime			
Thursday	Breakfast			
	Lunch			
	Dinner			
	Bedtime			
Friday	Breakfast			
	Lunch			
	Dinner			
	Bedtime			
Saturday	Breakfast			
	Lunch			
	Dinner			
	Bedtime			
Sunday	Breakfast			
	Lunch			
	Dinner			
	Bedtime			

Additional Notes

_____
_____
_____
_____
_____

Weekly Blood Sugar Log

Week_____

	Time	Before	After	Notes
Monday	Breakfast			
	Lunch			
	Dinner			
	Bedtime			
Tuesday	Breakfast			
	Lunch			
	Dinner			
	Bedtime			
Wednesday	Breakfast			
	Lunch			
	Dinner			
	Bedtime			
Thursday	Breakfast			
	Lunch			
	Dinner			
	Bedtime			
Friday	Breakfast			
	Lunch			
	Dinner			
	Bedtime			
Saturday	Breakfast			
	Lunch			
	Dinner			
	Bedtime			
Sunday	Breakfast			
	Lunch			
	Dinner			
	Bedtime			

Additional Notes

_____

_____

_____

_____

_____

Weekly Blood Sugar Log

Week_____

	Time	Before	After	Notes
Monday	Breakfast			
	Lunch			
	Dinner			
	Bedtime			
Tuesday	Breakfast			
	Lunch			
	Dinner			
	Bedtime			
Wednesday	Breakfast			
	Lunch			
	Dinner			
	Bedtime			
Thursday	Breakfast			
	Lunch			
	Dinner			
	Bedtime			
Friday	Breakfast			
	Lunch			
	Dinner			
	Bedtime			
Saturday	Breakfast			
	Lunch			
	Dinner			
	Bedtime			
Sunday	Breakfast			
	Lunch			
	Dinner			
	Bedtime			

Additional Notes

_____

_____

_____

_____

_____

Weekly Blood Sugar Log

Week_____

	Time	Before	After	Notes
Monday	Breakfast			
	Lunch			
	Dinner			
	Bedtime			
Tuesday	Breakfast			
	Lunch			
	Dinner			
	Bedtime			
Wednesday	Breakfast			
	Lunch			
	Dinner			
	Bedtime			
Thursday	Breakfast			
	Lunch			
	Dinner			
	Bedtime			
Friday	Breakfast			
	Lunch			
	Dinner			
	Bedtime			
Saturday	Breakfast			
	Lunch			
	Dinner			
	Bedtime			
Sunday	Breakfast			
	Lunch			
	Dinner			
	Bedtime			

Additional Notes

_____

_____

_____

_____

_____

Weekly Blood Sugar Log

Week_____

	Time	Before	After	Notes
Monday	Breakfast			
	Lunch			
	Dinner			
	Bedtime			
Tuesday	Breakfast			
	Lunch			
	Dinner			
	Bedtime			
Wednesday	Breakfast			
	Lunch			
	Dinner			
	Bedtime			
Thursday	Breakfast			
	Lunch			
	Dinner			
	Bedtime			
Friday	Breakfast			
	Lunch			
	Dinner			
	Bedtime			
Saturday	Breakfast			
	Lunch			
	Dinner			
	Bedtime			
Sunday	Breakfast			
	Lunch			
	Dinner			
	Bedtime			

Additional Notes

_____

_____

_____

_____

_____

Weekly Blood Sugar Log

Week_____

	Time	Before	After	Notes
Monday	Breakfast			
	Lunch			
	Dinner			
	Bedtime			
Tuesday	Breakfast			
	Lunch			
	Dinner			
	Bedtime			
Wednesday	Breakfast			
	Lunch			
	Dinner			
	Bedtime			
Thursday	Breakfast			
	Lunch			
	Dinner			
	Bedtime			
Friday	Breakfast			
	Lunch			
	Dinner			
	Bedtime			
Saturday	Breakfast			
	Lunch			
	Dinner			
	Bedtime			
Sunday	Breakfast			
	Lunch			
	Dinner			
	Bedtime			

Additional Notes

_____

_____

_____

_____

_____

Weekly Blood Sugar Log

Week_____

	Time	Before	After	Notes
Monday	Breakfast			
	Lunch			
	Dinner			
	Bedtime			
Tuesday	Breakfast			
	Lunch			
	Dinner			
	Bedtime			
Wednesday	Breakfast			
	Lunch			
	Dinner			
	Bedtime			
Thursday	Breakfast			
	Lunch			
	Dinner			
	Bedtime			
Friday	Breakfast			
	Lunch			
	Dinner			
	Bedtime			
Saturday	Breakfast			
	Lunch			
	Dinner			
	Bedtime			
Sunday	Breakfast			
	Lunch			
	Dinner			
	Bedtime			

Additional Notes

_____

_____

_____

_____

_____

Weekly Blood Sugar Log

Week_____

	Time	Before	After	Notes
Monday	Breakfast			
	Lunch			
	Dinner			
	Bedtime			
Tuesday	Breakfast			
	Lunch			
	Dinner			
	Bedtime			
Wednesday	Breakfast			
	Lunch			
	Dinner			
	Bedtime			
Thursday	Breakfast			
	Lunch			
	Dinner			
	Bedtime			
Friday	Breakfast			
	Lunch			
	Dinner			
	Bedtime			
Saturday	Breakfast			
	Lunch			
	Dinner			
	Bedtime			
Sunday	Breakfast			
	Lunch			
	Dinner			
	Bedtime			

Additional Notes

_____
_____
_____
_____
_____

Weekly Blood Sugar Log

Week_____

	Time	Before	After	Notes
Monday	Breakfast			
	Lunch			
	Dinner			
	Bedtime			
Tuesday	Breakfast			
	Lunch			
	Dinner			
	Bedtime			
Wednesday	Breakfast			
	Lunch			
	Dinner			
	Bedtime			
Thursday	Breakfast			
	Lunch			
	Dinner			
	Bedtime			
Friday	Breakfast			
	Lunch			
	Dinner			
	Bedtime			
Saturday	Breakfast			
	Lunch			
	Dinner			
	Bedtime			
Sunday	Breakfast			
	Lunch			
	Dinner			
	Bedtime			

Additional Notes

_____

_____

_____

_____

_____

Weekly Blood Sugar Log

Week_____

	Time	Before	After	Notes
Monday	Breakfast			
	Lunch			
	Dinner			
	Bedtime			
Tuesday	Breakfast			
	Lunch			
	Dinner			
	Bedtime			
Wednesday	Breakfast			
	Lunch			
	Dinner			
	Bedtime			
Thursday	Breakfast			
	Lunch			
	Dinner			
	Bedtime			
Friday	Breakfast			
	Lunch			
	Dinner			
	Bedtime			
Saturday	Breakfast			
	Lunch			
	Dinner			
	Bedtime			
Sunday	Breakfast			
	Lunch			
	Dinner			
	Bedtime			

Additional Notes

_____

_____

_____

_____

_____

Weekly Blood Sugar Log

Week_____

	Time	Before	After	Notes
Monday	Breakfast			
	Lunch			
	Dinner			
	Bedtime			
Tuesday	Breakfast			
	Lunch			
	Dinner			
	Bedtime			
Wednesday	Breakfast			
	Lunch			
	Dinner			
	Bedtime			
Thursday	Breakfast			
	Lunch			
	Dinner			
	Bedtime			
Friday	Breakfast			
	Lunch			
	Dinner			
	Bedtime			
Saturday	Breakfast			
	Lunch			
	Dinner			
	Bedtime			
Sunday	Breakfast			
	Lunch			
	Dinner			
	Bedtime			

Additional Notes

_____
_____
_____
_____
_____

Weekly Blood Sugar Log

Week_____

	Time	Before	After	Notes
Monday	Breakfast			
	Lunch			
	Dinner			
	Bedtime			
Tuesday	Breakfast			
	Lunch			
	Dinner			
	Bedtime			
Wednesday	Breakfast			
	Lunch			
	Dinner			
	Bedtime			
Thursday	Breakfast			
	Lunch			
	Dinner			
	Bedtime			
Friday	Breakfast			
	Lunch			
	Dinner			
	Bedtime			
Saturday	Breakfast			
	Lunch			
	Dinner			
	Bedtime			
Sunday	Breakfast			
	Lunch			
	Dinner			
	Bedtime			

Additional Notes

_____

_____

_____

_____

_____

Weekly Blood Sugar Log

Week_____

	Time	Before	After	Notes
Monday	Breakfast			
	Lunch			
	Dinner			
	Bedtime			
Tuesday	Breakfast			
	Lunch			
	Dinner			
	Bedtime			
Wednesday	Breakfast			
	Lunch			
	Dinner			
	Bedtime			
Thursday	Breakfast			
	Lunch			
	Dinner			
	Bedtime			
Friday	Breakfast			
	Lunch			
	Dinner			
	Bedtime			
Saturday	Breakfast			
	Lunch			
	Dinner			
	Bedtime			
Sunday	Breakfast			
	Lunch			
	Dinner			
	Bedtime			

Additional Notes

_____

_____

_____

_____

_____

Weekly Blood Sugar Log

Week_____

	Time	Before	After	Notes
Monday	Breakfast			
	Lunch			
	Dinner			
	Bedtime			
Tuesday	Breakfast			
	Lunch			
	Dinner			
	Bedtime			
Wednesday	Breakfast			
	Lunch			
	Dinner			
	Bedtime			
Thursday	Breakfast			
	Lunch			
	Dinner			
	Bedtime			
Friday	Breakfast			
	Lunch			
	Dinner			
	Bedtime			
Saturday	Breakfast			
	Lunch			
	Dinner			
	Bedtime			
Sunday	Breakfast			
	Lunch			
	Dinner			
	Bedtime			

Additional Notes

_____

_____

_____

_____

_____

Weekly Blood Sugar Log

Week_____

	Time	Before	After	Notes
Monday	Breakfast			
	Lunch			
	Dinner			
	Bedtime			
Tuesday	Breakfast			
	Lunch			
	Dinner			
	Bedtime			
Wednesday	Breakfast			
	Lunch			
	Dinner			
	Bedtime			
Thursday	Breakfast			
	Lunch			
	Dinner			
	Bedtime			
Friday	Breakfast			
	Lunch			
	Dinner			
	Bedtime			
Saturday	Breakfast			
	Lunch			
	Dinner			
	Bedtime			
Sunday	Breakfast			
	Lunch			
	Dinner			
	Bedtime			

Additional Notes

_____

_____

_____

_____

_____

Weekly Blood Sugar Log

Week_____

	Time	Before	After	Notes
Monday	Breakfast			
	Lunch			
	Dinner			
	Bedtime			
Tuesday	Breakfast			
	Lunch			
	Dinner			
	Bedtime			
Wednesday	Breakfast			
	Lunch			
	Dinner			
	Bedtime			
Thursday	Breakfast			
	Lunch			
	Dinner			
	Bedtime			
Friday	Breakfast			
	Lunch			
	Dinner			
	Bedtime			
Saturday	Breakfast			
	Lunch			
	Dinner			
	Bedtime			
Sunday	Breakfast			
	Lunch			
	Dinner			
	Bedtime			

Additional Notes

_____

_____

_____

_____

_____

Weekly Blood Sugar Log

Week_____

	Time	Before	After	Notes
Monday	Breakfast			
	Lunch			
	Dinner			
	Bedtime			
Tuesday	Breakfast			
	Lunch			
	Dinner			
	Bedtime			
Wednesday	Breakfast			
	Lunch			
	Dinner			
	Bedtime			
Thursday	Breakfast			
	Lunch			
	Dinner			
	Bedtime			
Friday	Breakfast			
	Lunch			
	Dinner			
	Bedtime			
Saturday	Breakfast			
	Lunch			
	Dinner			
	Bedtime			
Sunday	Breakfast			
	Lunch			
	Dinner			
	Bedtime			

Additional Notes

_____

_____

_____

_____

_____

Weekly Blood Sugar Log

Week_____

	Time	Before	After	Notes
Monday	Breakfast			
	Lunch			
	Dinner			
	Bedtime			
Tuesday	Breakfast			
	Lunch			
	Dinner			
	Bedtime			
Wednesday	Breakfast			
	Lunch			
	Dinner			
	Bedtime			
Thursday	Breakfast			
	Lunch			
	Dinner			
	Bedtime			
Friday	Breakfast			
	Lunch			
	Dinner			
	Bedtime			
Saturday	Breakfast			
	Lunch			
	Dinner			
	Bedtime			
Sunday	Breakfast			
	Lunch			
	Dinner			
	Bedtime			

Additional Notes

_____

_____

_____

_____

_____

Weekly Blood Sugar Log

Week_____

	Time	Before	After	Notes
Monday	Breakfast			
	Lunch			
	Dinner			
	Bedtime			
Tuesday	Breakfast			
	Lunch			
	Dinner			
	Bedtime			
Wednesday	Breakfast			
	Lunch			
	Dinner			
	Bedtime			
Thursday	Breakfast			
	Lunch			
	Dinner			
	Bedtime			
Friday	Breakfast			
	Lunch			
	Dinner			
	Bedtime			
Saturday	Breakfast			
	Lunch			
	Dinner			
	Bedtime			
Sunday	Breakfast			
	Lunch			
	Dinner			
	Bedtime			

Additional Notes

_____

_____

_____

_____

_____

Weekly Blood Sugar Log

Week_____

	Time	Before	After	Notes
Monday	Breakfast			
	Lunch			
	Dinner			
	Bedtime			
Tuesday	Breakfast			
	Lunch			
	Dinner			
	Bedtime			
Wednesday	Breakfast			
	Lunch			
	Dinner			
	Bedtime			
Thursday	Breakfast			
	Lunch			
	Dinner			
	Bedtime			
Friday	Breakfast			
	Lunch			
	Dinner			
	Bedtime			
Saturday	Breakfast			
	Lunch			
	Dinner			
	Bedtime			
Sunday	Breakfast			
	Lunch			
	Dinner			
	Bedtime			

Additional Notes

_____

_____

_____

_____

_____

Weekly Blood Sugar Log

Week_____

	Time	Before	After	Notes
Monday	Breakfast			
	Lunch			
	Dinner			
	Bedtime			
Tuesday	Breakfast			
	Lunch			
	Dinner			
	Bedtime			
Wednesday	Breakfast			
	Lunch			
	Dinner			
	Bedtime			
Thursday	Breakfast			
	Lunch			
	Dinner			
	Bedtime			
Friday	Breakfast			
	Lunch			
	Dinner			
	Bedtime			
Saturday	Breakfast			
	Lunch			
	Dinner			
	Bedtime			
Sunday	Breakfast			
	Lunch			
	Dinner			
	Bedtime			

Additional Notes

_____

_____

_____

_____

_____

Weekly Blood Sugar Log

Week_____

	Time	Before	After	Notes
Monday	Breakfast			
	Lunch			
	Dinner			
	Bedtime			
Tuesday	Breakfast			
	Lunch			
	Dinner			
	Bedtime			
Wednesday	Breakfast			
	Lunch			
	Dinner			
	Bedtime			
Thursday	Breakfast			
	Lunch			
	Dinner			
	Bedtime			
Friday	Breakfast			
	Lunch			
	Dinner			
	Bedtime			
Saturday	Breakfast			
	Lunch			
	Dinner			
	Bedtime			
Sunday	Breakfast			
	Lunch			
	Dinner			
	Bedtime			

Additional Notes

_____

_____

_____

_____

_____

Weekly Blood Sugar Log

Week_____

	Time	Before	After	Notes
Monday	Breakfast			
	Lunch			
	Dinner			
	Bedtime			
Tuesday	Breakfast			
	Lunch			
	Dinner			
	Bedtime			
Wednesday	Breakfast			
	Lunch			
	Dinner			
	Bedtime			
Thursday	Breakfast			
	Lunch			
	Dinner			
	Bedtime			
Friday	Breakfast			
	Lunch			
	Dinner			
	Bedtime			
Saturday	Breakfast			
	Lunch			
	Dinner			
	Bedtime			
Sunday	Breakfast			
	Lunch			
	Dinner			
	Bedtime			

Additional Notes

_____

_____

_____

_____

_____

Weekly Blood Sugar Log

Week_____

	Time	Before	After	Notes
Monday	Breakfast			
	Lunch			
	Dinner			
	Bedtime			
Tuesday	Breakfast			
	Lunch			
	Dinner			
	Bedtime			
Wednesday	Breakfast			
	Lunch			
	Dinner			
	Bedtime			
Thursday	Breakfast			
	Lunch			
	Dinner			
	Bedtime			
Friday	Breakfast			
	Lunch			
	Dinner			
	Bedtime			
Saturday	Breakfast			
	Lunch			
	Dinner			
	Bedtime			
Sunday	Breakfast			
	Lunch			
	Dinner			
	Bedtime			

Additional Notes

Weekly Blood Sugar Log

Week_____

	Time	Before	After	Notes
Monday	Breakfast			
	Lunch			
	Dinner			
	Bedtime			
Tuesday	Breakfast			
	Lunch			
	Dinner			
	Bedtime			
Wednesday	Breakfast			
	Lunch			
	Dinner			
	Bedtime			
Thursday	Breakfast			
	Lunch			
	Dinner			
	Bedtime			
Friday	Breakfast			
	Lunch			
	Dinner			
	Bedtime			
Saturday	Breakfast			
	Lunch			
	Dinner			
	Bedtime			
Sunday	Breakfast			
	Lunch			
	Dinner			
	Bedtime			

Additional Notes

_____
_____
_____
_____
_____

Weekly Blood Sugar Log

Week_____

	Time	Before	After	Notes
Monday	Breakfast			
	Lunch			
	Dinner			
	Bedtime			
Tuesday	Breakfast			
	Lunch			
	Dinner			
	Bedtime			
Wednesday	Breakfast			
	Lunch			
	Dinner			
	Bedtime			
Thursday	Breakfast			
	Lunch			
	Dinner			
	Bedtime			
Friday	Breakfast			
	Lunch			
	Dinner			
	Bedtime			
Saturday	Breakfast			
	Lunch			
	Dinner			
	Bedtime			
Sunday	Breakfast			
	Lunch			
	Dinner			
	Bedtime			

Additional Notes

Weekly Blood Sugar Log

Week_____

	Time	Before	After	Notes
Monday	Breakfast			
	Lunch			
	Dinner			
	Bedtime			
Tuesday	Breakfast			
	Lunch			
	Dinner			
	Bedtime			
Wednesday	Breakfast			
	Lunch			
	Dinner			
	Bedtime			
Thursday	Breakfast			
	Lunch			
	Dinner			
	Bedtime			
Friday	Breakfast			
	Lunch			
	Dinner			
	Bedtime			
Saturday	Breakfast			
	Lunch			
	Dinner			
	Bedtime			
Sunday	Breakfast			
	Lunch			
	Dinner			
	Bedtime			

Additional Notes

_____
_____
_____
_____
_____

Thank you!

WE ARE GLAD THAT YOU PURCHASED OUR
BOOK!
PLEASE LET US KNOW HOW WE CAN IMPROVE IT!
YOUR FEEDBACK IS ESSENTIAL TO US.

Contact us at:

M log'Sin@gmail.com

JUST TITLE THE EMAIL 'CREATIVE' AND WE WILL

GIVE YOU SOME EXTRA SURPRISES!